MY YOGA ROUTINE

10 POSTURES TO BEGIN A LIFETIME YOGA PRACTICE

CELESTE HARDY

Bloomington, IN  Milton Keynes, UK

authorHOUSE®

AuthorHouse™
1663 Liberty Drive, Suite 200
Bloomington, IN 47403
www.authorhouse.com
Phone: 1-800-839-8640

AuthorHouse™ UK Ltd.
500 Avebury Boulevard
Central Milton Keynes, MK9 2BE
www.authorhouse.co.uk
Phone: 08001974150

First published by AuthorHouse 5/21/2007

ISBN: 978-1-4259-7542-5 (sc)

Library of Congress Control Number: 2006909641

Printed in the United States of America
Bloomington, Indiana

This book is printed on acid-free paper.

DEDICATIONS

To Paula Tepedino, my Yoga guru, who helped me to recognize and harness my chaotic energy.

To Barbara Anne Cerrache, my best friend, who has and continues to give me emotional shelter through my many storms.

To Armando Passarelli, my good and gentle friend, who passed, triumphantly, yet, too early, from his earthly life.

To Lisa Kievit, supervisor and friend, at the Summit Area YMCA in New Jersey, who gave me consideration and leave, to strive for a fulfilled life.

To my children, grandchildren, parents, brothers, and sister, who have given me the courage and motivation to write this book.

CONTENTS

INTRODUCTION

In the following ten postures (exercises), we will explore correct form, movement, variations, and benefits. Some postures will have some cautionary advice. Any posture can be attempted up to the point where it becomes painful or awkward. A professional Yoga teacher should be consulted to ask whether or not the posture is too difficult or advanced for your body's flexibility, at the present time. As with any exercise activity, if you have any concerns about your ability to conduct this routine, safely, please consult a doctor, for a physical exam. Variations have been included for more difficult postures. Yet, I consider this book to be at the beginning level.

Please read the passages in the Preliminary Reading before beginning your study and practice.

Yoga teachers will find this book to be a valuable tool for students as the directions are precise and clear and will allow the student to practice in-between classes.

BREATHING

In Yoga, breathing is very important. It flushes the muscles with oxygen allowing them to become flexible throughout the movement of the posture. Relaxed and open muscles free blood flow which encourages healthy muscles. Inhale and exhale through the nostrils with the abdomen relaxed. Exhale when exerting movement. Allow the body to breath at its own speed – to regulate your exertion. Relax if your breathing is too quick. Do not hold your breath. One inhale and exhale is referred to as 'one cycle'.

WARM-UPS

In doing any exercise, it always is good to stretch muscles. Sitting on the floor, rotate your feet, one at a time, one way, and, then, the other. This is done at the ankles, about five times to the right and to the left.

Standing with your feet, together, raise the arms, upward, toward the ceiling. Gently stretch arms from the sockets of the shoulders. Feel the stretch through the elbow, wrists, into the fingertips. Exhale while lowering arms. This action will encourage flexibility. Repeat three times.

From a standing position, gently, lower the hands to the floor while relaxing shoulders. Tuck the chin in, slightly, and relax the neck. Legs can be bent or straight, depending on flexibility. While returning to a standing position, press into the soles, tighten the buttocks, and roll up, vertebra by vertebra. This action will increase the flexibility of the torso.

To warm up for many of the floor postures, we will be using what really are three postures in a sequence (what I refer to as Table, Dog, and Cat). We will do three sets.

We start on our hands and knees, head facing the floor, heels of the palms directly under the shoulder, and knees directly under the hips. Our fingers are spread, imagining that they are webbed, middle finger pointing forward. We must think of our fingers and palms as one block of support-spreading the palm just as we spread the ball pad of the sole when we are pressing the foot flat for support. The tops of our feet are extended from the ankle to the toe on the floor, resting, gently. To move from Table into Dog, we raise our head to look straight ahead, pushing our chin forward. Our eyes roll up to look at the ceiling, relaxing the abdomen, and letting it sag into an arc as we lift the tailbone up toward the ceiling. Gently, press down straightened arms into the palms, and, relaxing the abdomen, start three cycles of breathe.

Lowering the head, come back to Table, with eyes looking at the floor. Lift shoulders and back into an arc like a frightened Cat, pressing, gently, into palms. Tuck the tailbone, under, and bring forehead down, looking through legs toward the tailbone, lengthen neck, so that the crown of the head goes toward the floor. Relax the abdomen, inhale, and let the body count three cycles while you observe and focus on your breathing. Come out and repeat the sequence two more times.

The benefit of this sequence is a more limber spine and stronger arms and shoulders as well as more relaxed lower back.

WARM-UPS (cont.)

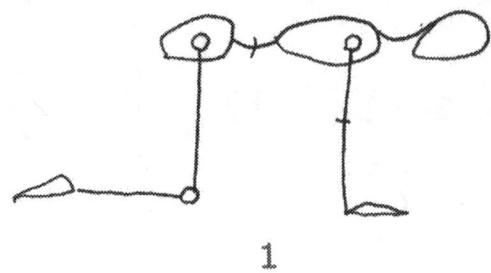

1

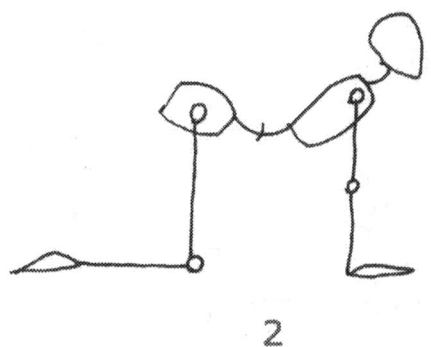

2

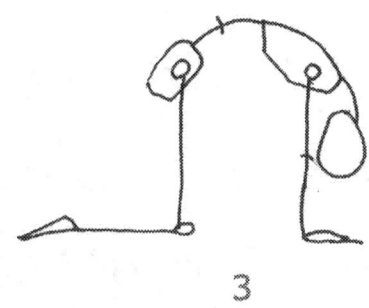

3

THE ABDOMEN

When you think of the abdominal cavity, you are visualizing a large, soft area containing internal organs covered by skin. It starts from the triangular arch in the ribs to the high points of the pelvis down to the pubic bone.

Relax all the muscles, fully and gently, within the entire oval of the abdomen. You will notice an immediate intake of air – an inhale; then, an exhale. Although you start the breathing process, voluntarily, after the first inhale, the body will take over. Let it. Just observe the pace (speed) of the rhythm (shallow or deep). This is a good indicator of whether you should 'relax' or 'increase your effort'. It is good to breathe, gently and evenly, throughout the entire workout. Do not hold your breath. Oxygen will energize and heal the muscles.

RESTING POSTURES

There are two resting postures that we will be employing in this book. The first is Dead Man's Posture which is described in Section Ten. The other posture, I will refer to as Leaf.

To assume Leaf, come down from Table, bend the knees, bring the toes, together, then, move the knees, out as far as is possible, comfortably. Bring the buttocks back as close to the heels, as possible. Extend the arms, forward, and rest on the floor as you open the hands, bring the chest down (coming down closer to the ground with the elbows touching and lengthening the arms along the floor, even more). Rest.

Opening the legs enables the abdomen to be relaxed with nothing pushing against it. Allow yourself to relax and breath, evenly and gently, for about a minute, circling attention to your body's muscles from the toes of one foot through the legs, trunk, head, arms, down the other leg to the toes, relaxing every tense muscle you encounter. Imagine that you are exhaling through each of those muscles. Rest. Clear any tension from your head and face. Breath.

RESTING POSTURES 1 & 2

Note: the first Resting Posture is LEAF, as illustrated, below. The second resting posture is Dead Man's Posture. Refer to its illustration in Section Ten.

LEAF

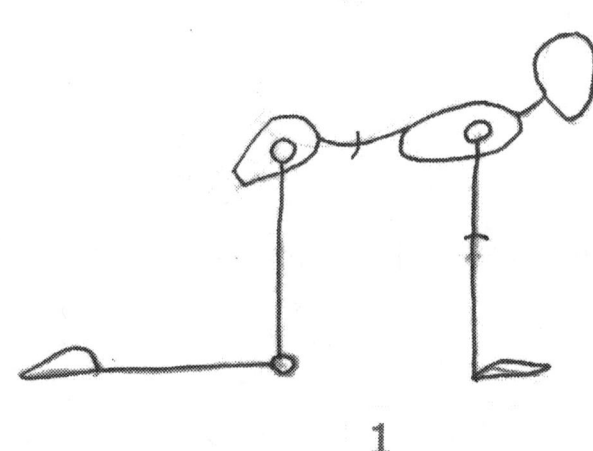

1

2

THE EDGE

You will see me refer to 'the edge' many times throughout this book. 'The edge' is the farthest stretch to which you can push your muscles without pain. REMEMBER THIS: Do not push into pain or strain, and breath (to prevent injury to the circulatory system and the muscles).

A PRACTICE SESSION

A good practice session is, for a beginner, around a half-hour. Yet, even if you only have five minutes, if you are focused, it will be a beneficial time spent. What matters is consistency and dedication. Yoga can be done anywhere, anytime. It can be done, sitting in an office chair, hanging on a strap in the subway, or changing a diaper. It is harmony of body, mind, and spirit – relaxing muscles, tensing others, and moving with assurance.

SETS

When you begin practicing Yoga, it is more important to work on perfecting the form rather than doing the postures, many times. So, start with one or two sets and build up, slowly, over time.

LEVELS

Different variations are illustrated in certain postures to give you an opportunity to do the posture at your own level of strength. Move from the first level, upward. Never move on until you feel confident of the level you are practicing.

PROPS

You may wish to purchase a mat to practice Yoga. Also, for certain postures it is advisable to have a good blanket. Yoga shops, health food stores (like Whole Foods), and, sometimes, sport stores sell mats and blankets. If you cannot find one, a tightly-woven blanket will do. It should be folded and pressed smooth with no bumps in order to support the head or to do some floor postures where there could be pain associated with contact with the floor.

HANDS AND FEET AS SUPPORT

There are postures that depend on the feet and hands for support. The hands in Table, for example, must have a flat palm and fingers outstretched (as though webbed). The palms and fingers should be thought of us one unit and weight should be pressed upon, evenly. The feet should do the same – the toes, spread, the ball of the foot, flat and firm, and the side and heel (not the instep), working together with all other parts, to make one firm, yet, gentle unit of support.

THINGS TO REMEMBER

_____

_____

_____

_____

_____

_____

_____

_____

_____

_____

SECTION ONE

MOUNTAIN

CAUTION: People with high blood pressure shouldn't hold their arms up straight over their heads for the full count of the posture. While others are holding for the full count, they can raise on an exhale and lower on an inhale for as many times as comfortable.

To begin:

From a standing position, the *feet* are from one to four inches apart (approximately), depending on body build. It is best to be balanced and anchored, firmly, yet, softly, on the ground. Feet are parallel (from in between the second and third toe, draw an imaginary line to the middle of each heel;

imagine both lines are parallel; then the feet will be parallel).

Gently lift the *kneecaps*, tighten the *thigh muscles* (quadriceps), tighten the *buttocks*, and tuck the *tailbone*, under, gently. Keep all muscles contracted, at this point.

KEEP GOING. Bring the *shoulder blades*, together, in the back as you lift the *chest*, slightly (to feel the chest open, brings arms up to shoulder level, lower shoulders down and roll back, lower arms to the side of the body). Keep this position as you relax the *shoulders* and the *abdomen*. Inhale and exhale through the *nostrils*. Look straight forward as you lift the *crown* of the *head* to the ceiling, keeping face forward, relaxing the neck muscles. Now, gently, yet, firmly, press the feet into the ground (like a footprint in the sand), using the 'whole' sole.

Keeps your arms straight by your sides, shoulders relaxed. This is Level One. Level Two starts by bringing the arms from a straight side-of-the-body position, turning *palms* upward, to a straight upward position with *palms* touching (reaching toward the ceiling). Try to keep the *biceps* in line with and near the *ears*.

In both levels, pay attention to the breathing, by: relaxing the *abdomen* which, when done fully, will cause the *nostrils* immediately to inhale and exhale. Once you are comfortable with your breath, just observe it. Your body will breathe without your trying to control it. While holding the posture, count three inhales and exhales (three cycles). Then, lower the arms. Bring hands into prayer position, relax, and lower arms, to the sides.

This is your first set. You may wish to do two or three more sets *or* increase your 'cycle' count. If you feel no pain or discomfort, GO AHEAD.

REMEMBER: Level One is with arms hanging by the sides of the body. Level Two is with arms overhead (remember, if you have HIGH BLOOD PRESSURE and wish to attempt Level Two, in order to be safe, you must follow the CAUTION directions at the beginning of Section One).

I have underlined key words in this section because MOUNTAIN posture is a fundamental starting point of standing postures and should be mastered – the form along with proper breathing.

MOUNTAIN

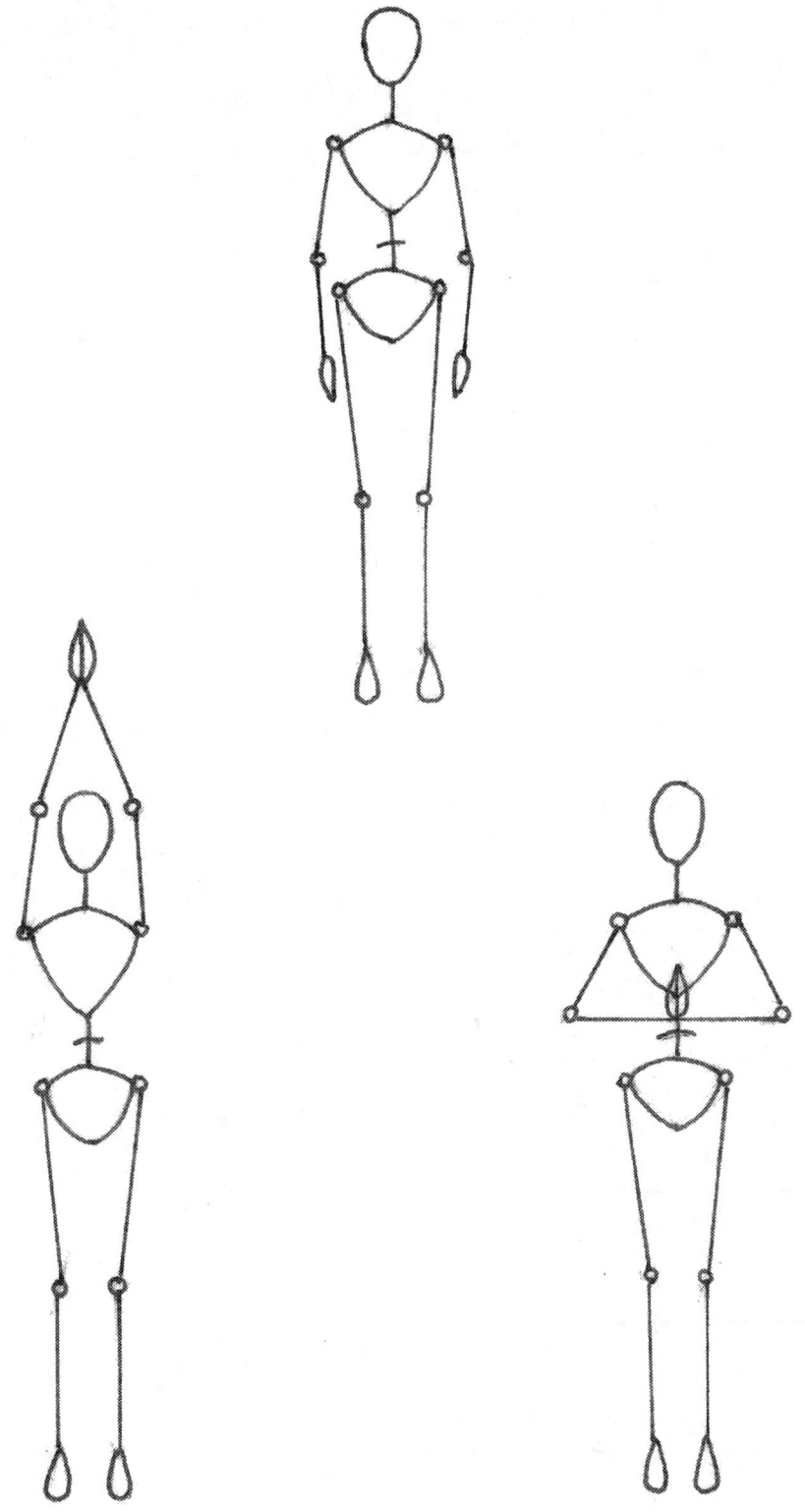

THINGS TO REMEMBER

_____

_____

_____

_____

_____

_____

_____

_____

_____

_____

SECTION TWO

TRIANGLE

Standing in mountain posture, sink the soles of the feet, evenly, into the mat or ground, feet together or slightly apart, depending on body build. Lift arms up and out to the sides at shoulder height and stretch them as though they are being pulled, gently, away from the sockets. Keep that gentle tension throughout the posture. Open the legs three to four feet apart. Keep feet pointing forward. Pivot the right foot on heel 90 degrees out to right side; pivot the left foot about 30 degrees in the same direction as the right foot. Gently, press into the soles of each foot (balance can be attained by keeping big toe and outside heel pressed down on each foot). Pull up the kneecaps, gently tightening the quadriceps (thigh muscles). With the buttocks muscles, pull the leg muscles up while pressing into the firmly planted, yet, evenly spread soles. At this point, keep the legs and body from the waist down, stationery. Move the upper body toward the side as though you are sliding the arms on a shoulder-level stone wall (look at illustration). Do not bend forward leg. If the knee bends, you are going to far to the side. When you have gone as far as you can – a good stretch to the edge, then, turn the arms, vertically (look at the illustration), turning like an airplane – one arm stretching toward the ceiling, one arm toward the floor. REMEMBER: hands are straight out of the wrists; fingers are straight out of the palms.

Bring the lower hand down touching the back of the calf muscle. If that is all the farther it can go, fine. Use this point to steady the arm if you go down, farther. If you can touch the floor, lay the hand flat (if possible) on the floor near the ankle.

NOW, YOU ARE IN THE MAJOR POSITION OF THE POSTURE.

Keep you torso facing forward throughout the whole count of holding the posture, as much as possible. This will help you focus and balance. Relax your abdomen, fully. When you do this, you will inhale, naturally. Relax and let your body breath. Observe the inhales and exhales. You should work up to ten cycles (remember, inhale and exhale are one cycle) in each held position. Yet, if you only can do one full cycle and you let your body do the breathing, then, you are doing what you should do and this is a GREAT START.

When you want to come out of the posture, come back to the upright position by using the strength of the back leg buttocks and leg muscles and pressing on the back sole (especially the heel) as one whole unit. Come up, drop arms, bring feet, together, and do the left side, starting from the Mountain Posture, going to the left.

Do one or two sets to begin; one to five cycles of breath while holding the final posture.

TRIANGLE

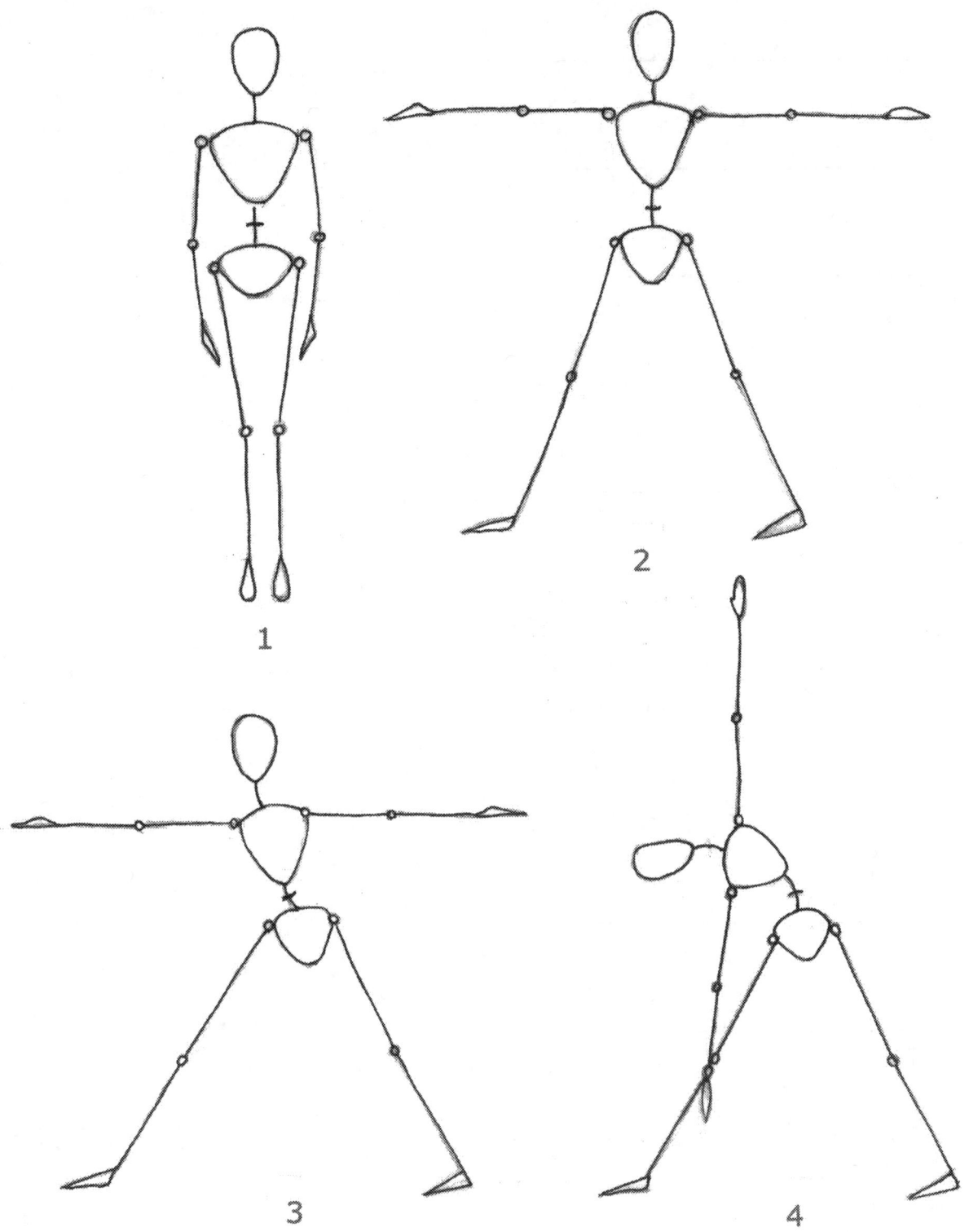

1

2

3

4

THINGS TO REMEMBER

_____

_____

_____

_____

_____

_____

_____

_____

_____

_____

SECTION THREE

CHAIR

CAUTION: In the third phase of the posture when hands are raised toward the ceiling, if you feel dizziness, labored breathing, or tightness in the chest, lower arms to second phase or come out of the posture, completely.

Chair is a dynamic posture. In order to do it, correctly, you must build from the ground up. There are many benefits. There is a wonderful extreme stretch and isometric aspect to the posture. It can alleviate backaches and help weak ankles, weak shoulders, and weak arms, by building muscle strength and giving more structural strength from joint to joint.

Chair has three phases (refer to illustration) and two levels. If you feel that you only can do the first for the time being, this is fine. Even at level one, the benefits are enormous.

Standing in Mountain Posture, staying erect, bend the knees until you feel the soles flatten and, your body naturally, stops. Then, extend the tailbone, outward, as though you are sitting on an imaginary chair. As you are doing this, raise your arms straight out in front of you, at shoulder level, parallel to each other and the floor, hands straight out from the arms, palms facing the floor. Keep the 'entire' sole of each foot anchored on the floor, pressing, evenly, without strain, from the toes and ball along the side to the heel. Do not press into the instep. This will prevent injury to the knee and will position you, properly. After relaxing the abdomen, hold the posture for five cycles. Do not force breathing – listen to the body. Breathe through the nostrils.

To move into the next level, tuck the tailbone under, gently, and raise the arms straight up toward the ceiling, attempting to bring the biceps as close (as possible) to the ears. Open the chest. Look straight forward. Breathe (five cycles). When finished, lower arms and press weight into the soles. Come back into Mountain.

At all times, during both levels of Chair, keep soles anchored, firmly, yet, gently, into the floor. Knees are over the instep of the feet. NOTE: I have had cartilage problems from an accident in high school gym class, many years, ago. I must not injure my knees. I can say with confidence that if you keep your soles pressed down, evenly, and do not lift the toes or heels, and, keep your tailbone extended outward and knees over the instep, there will be no problems. Always refer to the illustration.

The benefits of Chair are numerous from the feet up. The soles are stretched and muscles strengthened – the same with the calves and thighs. Tucking in the tailbone, whenever you are able, reduces stress on the lower back. Holding shoulders down and relaxed relieves neck strain. Holding arms in position, in both levels, produces strength and good alignment. Last of all, Chair teaches us to focus, breath evenly, and discipline one's nature.

CHAIR

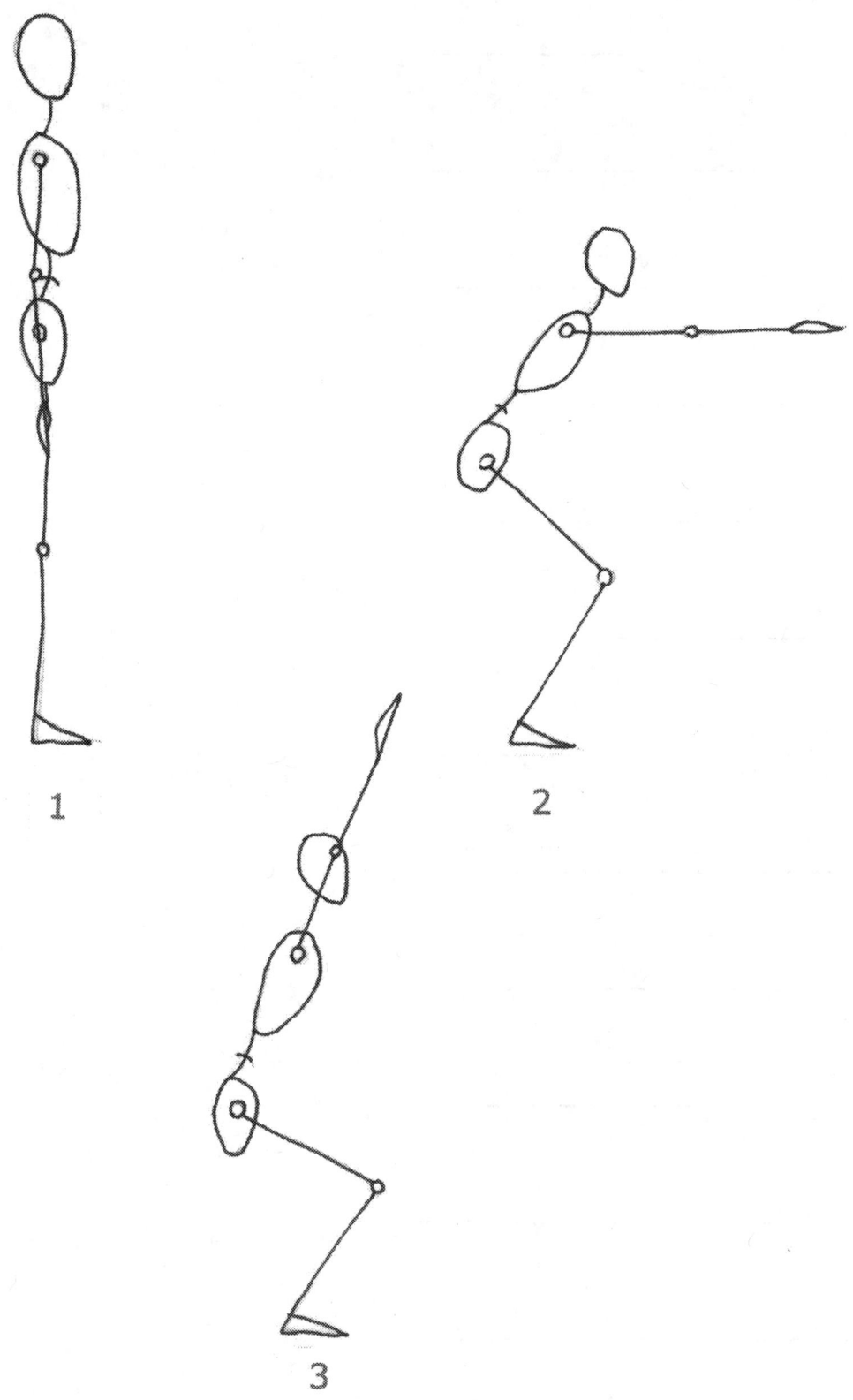

1

2

3

THINGS TO REMEMBER

_____

_____

_____

_____

_____

_____

_____

_____

_____

_____

SECTION FOUR

PLANK

Starting in Table (for a detailed description of proper form, refer to the Warm Up section), extended right leg, back, straight out, first, then, the left; put weight on the toes and ball of each foot as in a push-up. Lift the body as in the first phase of a push-up – straight arms and straight body with the exception that the neck, being in line with the rest of the spine, the head is facing forward the eyes are looking at the floor. The buttocks is kept down, accentuating the straight line of the posture.

The legs muscles are tightened as well as the buttocks, abdomen, and arm muscles. Contract, gently, while breathing through the nostrils for the duration of the posture. Think of the torso and the legs as one strong unit.

In each hand, the fingers are spread with middle fingers pointing straight forward and the palm is as flat as possible. Think of the fingers and palms as one unit of support and try to distribute the weight that the hands and feet are bearing throughout the body, evenly. The wrists may feel weak, at first, so you may want to do only one or two sets. Try to hold the posture between three to five full cycles of breath.

This posture may look quite effortless to the onlooker. It is deceiving. You may feel your abs tremble a little and your toes and wrists may be weak until they become used to the stretch and the bearing of the weight of the body. Tightening the buttocks and pulling up the muscles in the legs as well as tightening the shoulders and lifting the muscles in the arms will take pressure off of the feet and wrists. All of these adjustments will occur to you more and more throughout your practice if you are diligent and thoughtful.

The benefits are instantly obvious – more flexibility and strength in the feet and hands and abdominal area. The buttocks, shoulder muscles, arms, and legs will become increasingly stronger.

PLANK

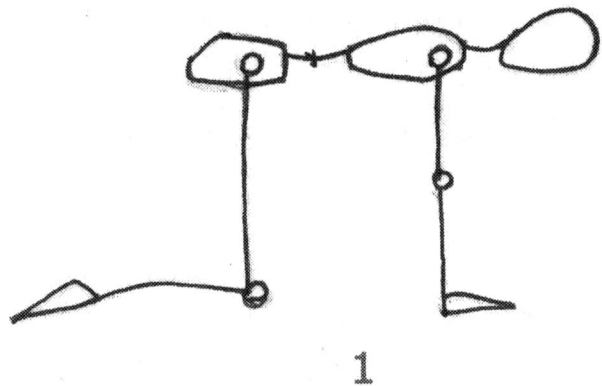

1

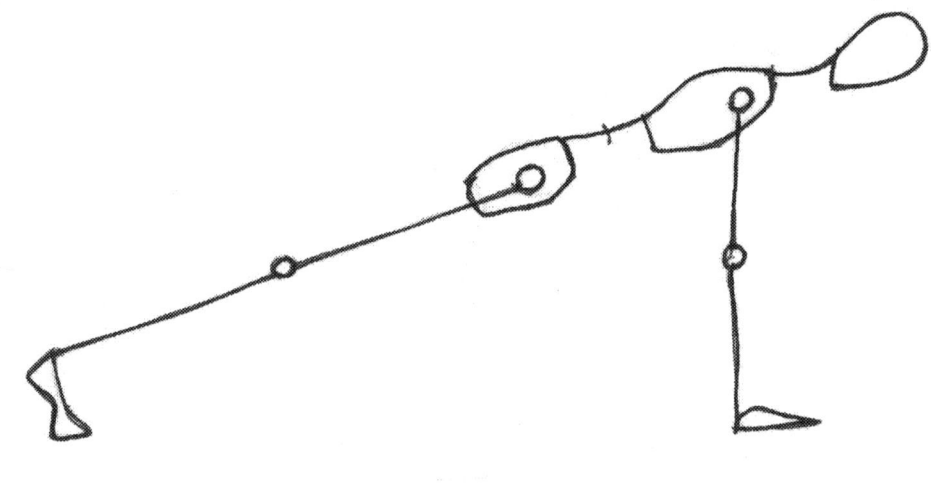

2

THINGS TO REMEMBER

_____

_____

_____

_____

_____

_____

_____

_____

_____

_____

SECTION FIVE

DOWNWARD FACING DOG

We begin in TABLE. Gently, bring your head down so that you are able to look through the legs. Come onto the balls of the feet. Gently, raise the tailbone toward the ceiling. Walk your hands forward one or two steps and adjust for comfort. Separate your feet, approximately four inches, keeping them parallel and somewhat in line with the hands. Hands are spread as though they are webbed with the middle fingers pointing, forward. The balls of the feet are spread, pressing down, firmly, and, evenly, as possible.

Open and extend the chest toward the shins, bringing the crown of the head toward the floor. The head and the hands will make a triangle. Keep opening the chest and moving it toward the shins. Now, the challenge is to hold the form and breathe. Keep the arms straight while flattening the palms, gently. Push the strength of the arms from the shoulders into the palms and think of the shoulders, arms, and hands as one strong unit. Relax and breathe, evenly.

Keeping the legs straight and the muscles tight, as possible, lower the heels to a comfortable position. To prevent injury, do not push into pain or strain the Achilles' tendon area. Bring the head toward the floor as far as possible. Now, pay attention to your breathing, through the nostrils, evenly.

Ideally, Downward Facing Dog should be held for five or more minutes. You may begin by observing your involuntary breathing for the count of ten cycles (ten inhales and exhales). Always remember, to keep the arms and legs as straight as possible. To straighten the arms, bring the elbows in toward the head, pushing, gently, into the palms. Keep breathing.

To come down, bring the knees, down. The toes come together. Bring the buttocks toward the heels and move the knees, as far as possible, comfortably, outward. Extend the arms forward, open the chest to the floor and bring the elbows onto the floor. The forehead rests on the mat. The arms are long and parallel. The open legs enable to torso to rest without the pressure of the thighs (this is especially beneficial for pregnant women and overweight people). You have seen this posture when a baby sleeps with the torso flat and legs drawn up.

DOWNWARD FACING DOG

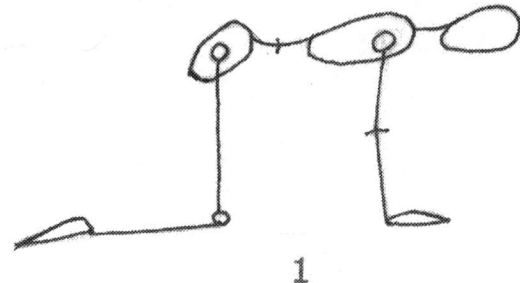

1

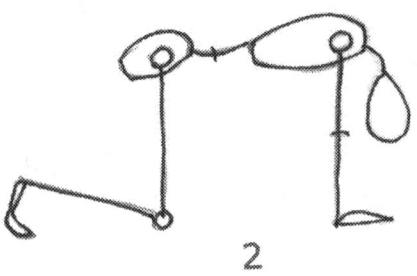

2

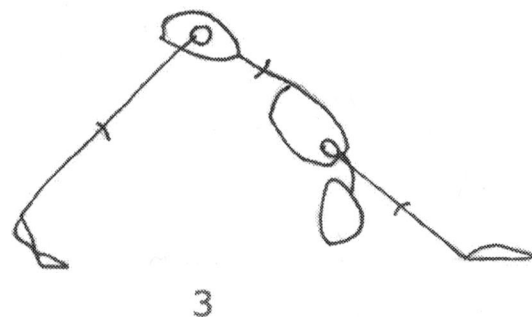

3

THINGS TO REMEMBER

_____

_____

_____

_____

_____

_____

_____

_____

_____

_____

SECTION SIX

UPWARD FACING DOG

Fold a blanket and place it on the floor where you can rest your chin, comfortably, on a flat one inch surface (the Mexican blankets sold in Yoga shops are ideal).

Starting in Table, extend both legs, backward, resting on the tops of your feet. Legs are off the ground with their weight being supported by the tops of the feet and straight arms with the flattened palms and spread fingers of the hands. The body is in a 'lean-to' position. Bring the chin forward, rolling the eyes up toward the ceiling.

Relax the torso, lowering abdomen toward the floor, opening chest and rolling shoulders back down.

Breath and hold up to three cycles if not in pain. This is Level One. This is an adequate routine for a beginner. If you wish to increase the stretch, you must pay particular attention to the neck to avoid injury.

Level Two of Upward Facing Dog will start in Table, tucking the tailbone under and holding a slight tension in the buttocks. After extending legs outward and lowering abdomen, you move into the arc, imagining a space between each vertebra starting at the bottom of the spine. Lengthen the back as you follow a gentle curve through the back and neck through the crown of the head. The space between each vertebra is long and follows the arc. Do not bend the head back. Keep it in its normal position on the neck following the line of the arc. When lifting the head, bring the shoulders down, so that the line is 'long and strong'. Hold a slight tension in the torso while opening the chest in the front and breathing, evenly.

Eyes look up to the ceiling. Fingers are spread and palms are flat on the mat, giving appropriate support to the body. Keep tension in the legs to keep the form and strengthen the legs.

Breath from three to five cycles of breath, letting the body's involuntary pace be the timing.

Be vigilant when coming out of the posture. Lower the body to the floor onto the belly. Rest the head to one side on the blanket with shoulders relaxing on the mat.

The benefits are: strengthened legs and arms; flexibility of the spine.

UPWARD FACING DOG

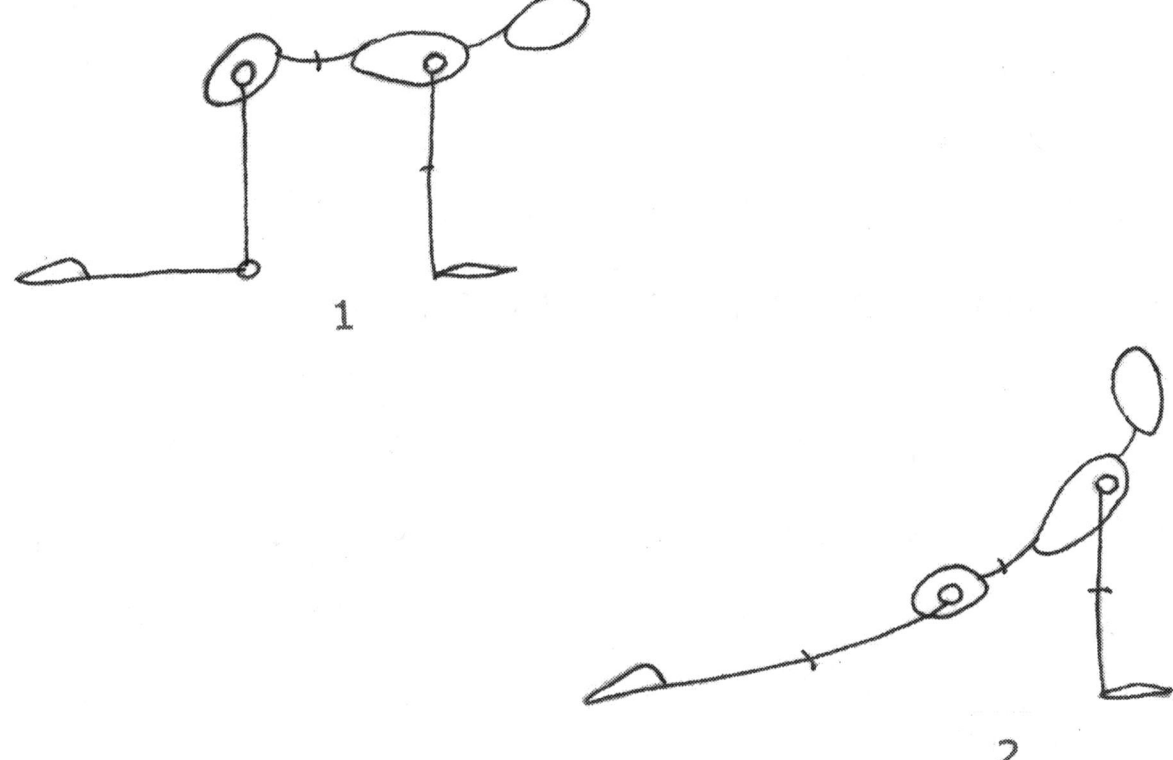

1

2

THINGS TO REMEMBER

_____

_____

_____

_____

_____

_____

_____

_____

_____

_____

SECTION SEVEN

COBRA

Cobra has three levels. The last one closely resembles Upward Facing Dog except that from the pubic bone through the legs and feet, the lower body is on the floor.

Have your blanket flattened and folded to a width of one inch. Rest the chin on the blanket and, then, turn the head on its side, alternating, from set to set.

Level One starts with belly down, arms are alongside the body. Bring the hands next to and in line with the breast line. Using the torso, without putting weight on the hands, gently, lift the body up on its power (like a snake raising its upper body off the ground) all the way to the pubic bone. Open the chest and relax the shoulders. The chin extends, slightly forward, lengthening the neck from the chin to the chest, gently. The arms are bent with the elbows close into the body. You will feel when the hands, naturally, engage the floor to support the weight of the body. Only then, press into the hands, push the pubic bone down, and, keeping the head straight forward, roll the eyes up toward the ceiling. Hold for three cycles of breath, holding the tension in the arms.

Level Two follows the same directions. The difference is that the starting position of the hands is about two inches down from the breast line, next to the body (mid-ribs). You will rise and find that you go up a little higher. Tensing the arms, spread palms and fingers. There will be a slight arc in the spine if you open the chest and lift upward. Let the neck vertebrae lengthen away from the shoulders. Do not bend the neck back. Bend the middle of the back and open the chest keeping the neck in line with the spine. Count three to five cycles of breath while holding. Make sure that the body's involuntary breathing is the count.

Note: Always be careful to imagine a straight line from between the shoulder blades to the crown of the head and keep the muscles long and tight as you keep in mind the line of the form (such as an arc) or going backward in line with the spine or coming forward out of a position back to the starting posture.

Come down onto the blanket and turn head to one side (shoulders should be off the blanket).

Level Three begins the same as did Level One and Two. The arms bend and are close to the end of the ribcage (near the waist). The hands spread . Again, the torso rises like a snake on its own power until the hands engage. Now, it is possible to straighten the arms by shrugging the shoulders. Extend the upper torso away from the lower torso. Press the pubic bone toward the floor and start the arc. Remember that the middle of the back through the crown is one unit. The eyes look toward the ceiling. DO NOT BEND THE NECK BACK. Inhale and start three to five cycles of breathe.

Come down, gently. Rest the arms by the sides or under the head with the head turned to the side.

The benefits of Cobra are: increased flexibility of the spine, stronger arms and hands, and increased oxygen flow to the lungs.

COBRA

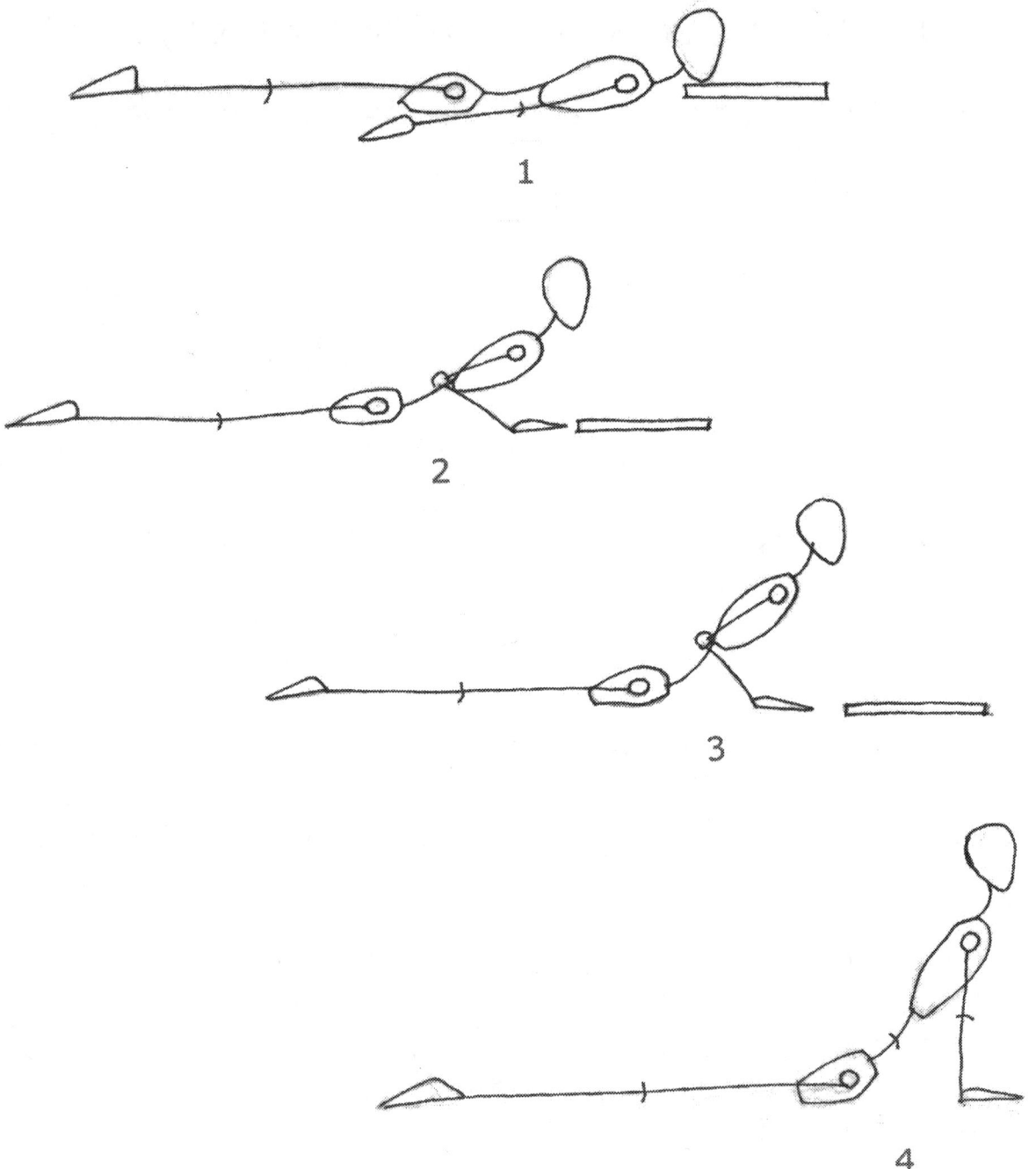

1

2

3

4

THINGS TO REMEMBER

_____

_____

_____

_____

_____

_____

_____

_____

_____

_____

SECTION EIGHT

BOW

Place a blanket in front of your head to use when resting your chin and when resting your head to the side when coming out of the posture into DEAD MAN'S POSTURE, at the end.

Rest your chin on the edge of the blanket. The arms are straight, next to the body. The whole body is resting, belly down, on the floor. Keeping the legs, together, raise the right lower leg, at the knee, toward the right buttocks. Hold the right ankle with the right hand. Bring the left lower leg up to the left buttocks, holding the left ankle with the left hand. At the same time, lift the torso up while holding the ankles, keeping the abdomen pressing into the floor, while lifting the legs. Open the chest and relax your shoulders. The eyes roll up and look at the ceiling while keeping the head in the same position, facing forward.

All body types are different: some of us have short legs and a long torso. Some of us have a short torso and long legs. You might find that one section is easier to raise than the other. Don't get discouraged. Keep doing your best. The benefits are enormous.

Hold the uplifted posture from one to five cycles of breath. Then lower legs and torso. Lower your arms to your sides. Turn the head to one side and rest. If this is really uncomfortable, you can bring your hands up under the head to support it. When you do more than one set, alternate the turning of your head to the other side. Your legs are together and long. Rest on the tops of the feet, stretched out.

There is an alternate way if you find BOW too difficult. Laying on your right side, bring the left leg bent back and hold the ankle with the left hand. Arch your back to make the form of the BOW. Lengthen the neck from the shoulders and hold. You can balance the body by bringing the right arm forward and applying pressure on the floor. Hold one to five cycles of breath. Then, repeat on the left side, with the right leg, held by the right hand, and, supported by the straight left arm on the floor.

The benefits of both variations are: relaxation and flexibility of the neck and shoulder area and the strengthening of the spine, buttocks, and legs.

BOW

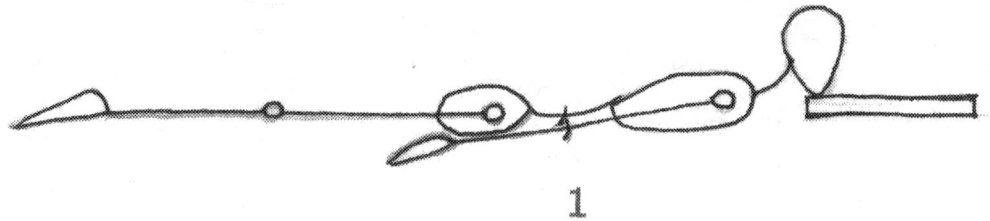

1

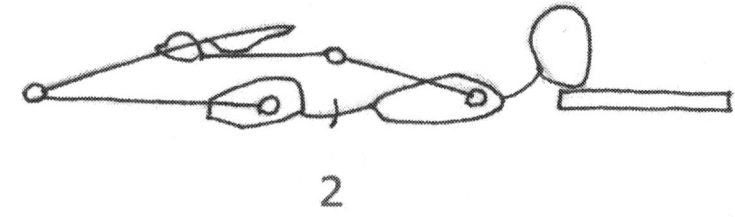

2

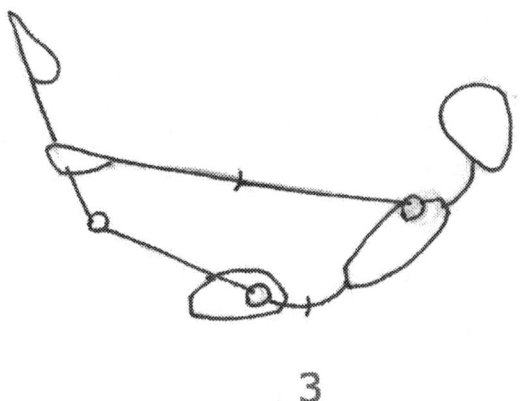

3

THINGS TO REMEMBER

_____

_____

_____

_____

_____

_____

_____

_____

_____

_____

SECTION NINE

SIDE FLOOR TWISTS

Now, we begin the cool down phase of our workout. Laying on our back, place the head on the edge of the flattened blanket. Press the chin into the area of the sternum's notch (the area at the bottom of the neck which resembles a small gully). Lengthen the back of the neck to protect it. The shoulders are on the mat. The arms are by our sides. Walk the feet up toward the buttocks, press into the soles, and raise up the buttocks. Lower the back down, again, while pressing on the middle of the back all the way to the tailbone to settle into a flat back, flush with the ground.

Raise both knees, up, to the chest, keeping the legs, together. Hold the right knee with the right hand and the left knee with the left hand. Gently, press both knees toward the chest. Hold the legs, there, while you raise the arms straight towards the ceiling about ten inches apart, palm facing palm. Then, bring the arms straight out to the sides making a T configuration.

Bring the legs over to the floor to the right, relax left hip, shoulder, arm, and feet. The palms are facing the ceiling. Turn the head toward the left hand and relax the body as much as possible. Breathing, even, through the nostrils, relax the abdomen. Relax the fingers and toes. Count about ten cycles of breath. Bring the head back to the center, looking at the ceiling. Brings the legs back to the chest and swing them, gently, to the left side, to the floor. Relax the right hip, shoulder, arm, and feet. Turn the head toward the right hand and relax. Relax the fingers and the toes. Now, breath, evenly – about ten cycles.

Bring the head back to the center. Bring the legs up and back to the center. The hands come back, right hand holding right knee and left hand holding left knee. Release the hands and bring the arms alongside, yet, slightly, away from the body in an A configuration. Lower the legs, out, one at a time, to the floor, next to each other. Turn the feet out, keeping the heels, together. Turn the palms, upward. The chin rests in the sternum's notch, as before. Relax the shoulders, fingers, and toes.

After having rested about thirty seconds, if you wish to repeat the posture, go through all the steps, as before.

The benefits are: lengthening and relaxing of the spine increasing circulation and flexibility; an exercise in learning the technique of gentle relaxation to increase alertness and positive attitude.

SIDE FLOOR TWISTS

(cool down)

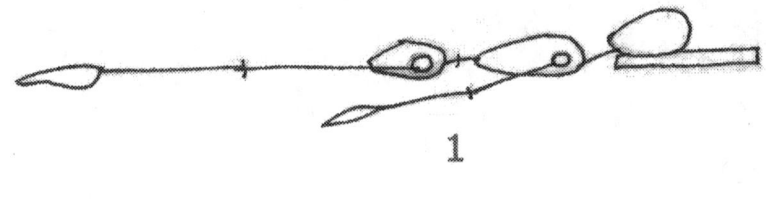

1

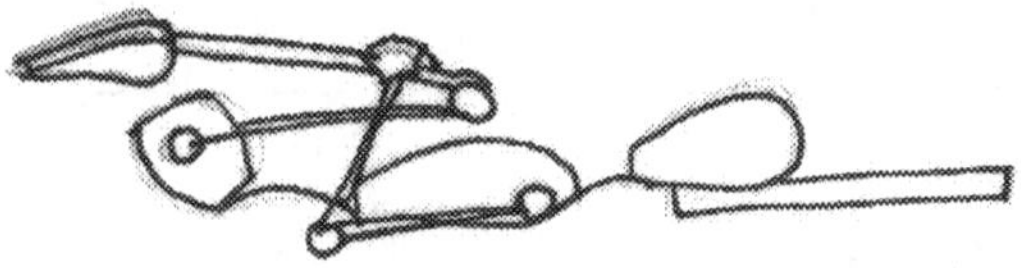

2

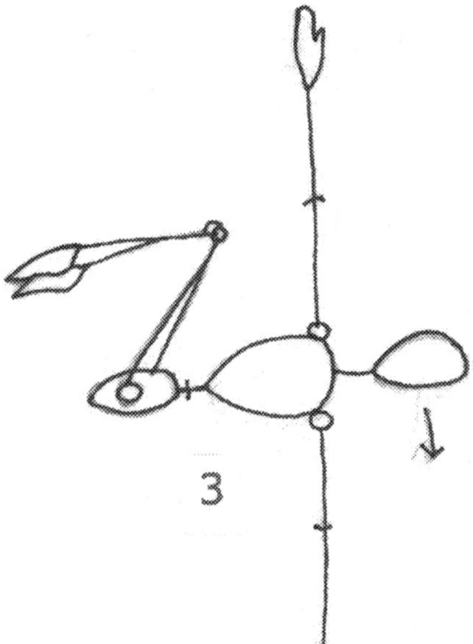

3

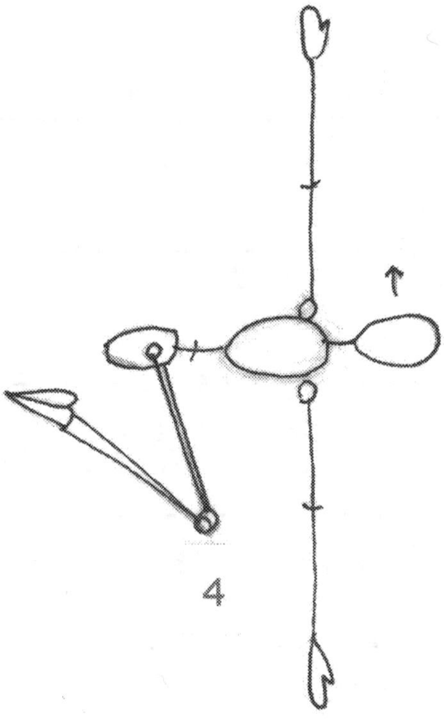

4

THINGS TO REMEMBER

_____

_____

_____

_____

_____

_____

_____

_____

_____

_____

SECTION TEN

DEAD MAN'S POSTURE

Place the blanket to support the neck and head. With the shoulders resting on the floor, stretch the back as flat as possible on the mat, and bring the legs, together. Bring the heels, together, or a few inches apart and turn the feet outward and relax. Tuck the tailbone under and relax the back. Place the arms, long, by the sides of the body, yet, slightly, apart (the trunk and arms in the form of an A).

The body is resting. Stretch the fingers and toes to get out any stiffness. Starting from the feet, relax each portion of the body: the calves, thighs, lower back, buttocks, and arms. Imagine that you are exhaling through every muscle from the bottom to the top.

Smile to relax muscles in the lower face. Shrug the forehead to relax those muscles and soften the eyes to relax the muscles in the eye sockets.

Allow your thoughts to drift like clouds. This is your settling posture, the posture which ends your practice. Relax the abdomen and focus on your 'breath', observing the feelings of your entire body. If you have a blanket, nearby, you may want to cover yourself or have a friend do it for you, wrapping the blanket around your feet to feel as warm and comfortable as possible.

Try to imagine you are going to sleep, yet staying awake. Rest and breath. There probably is not a more relaxing posture on earth. Enjoy!

DEAD MAN'S POSTURE

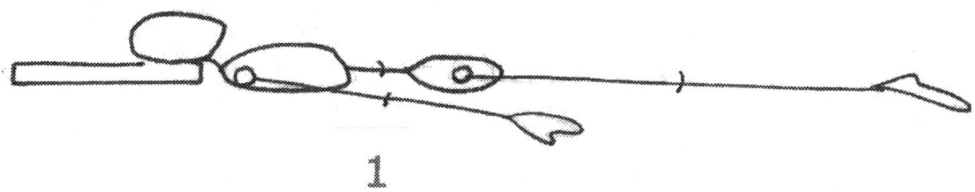

1

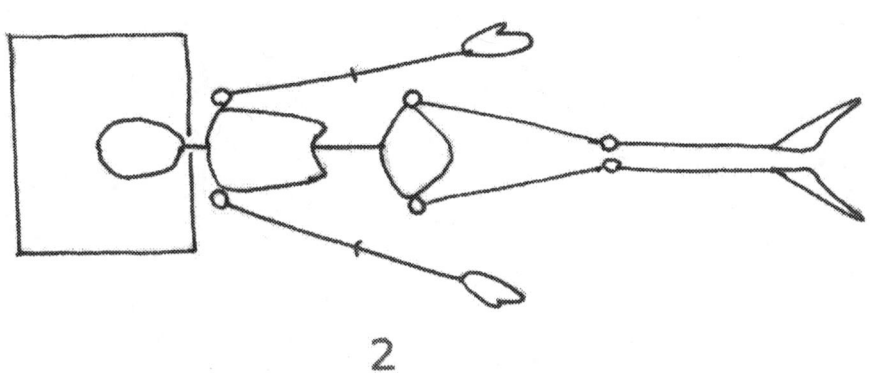

2

CONCLUSION

Well, those are our postures. I hope that you will read and reread the directions and create a program for yourself that will be fulfilling in your own personal practice.

Remember, don't be too critical, just dedicated and careful. That is the key to Yoga's harmony.

JOURNAL

_____

_____

_____

_____

_____

_____

_____

_____

_____